THE ART OF KETO AND FASTING FOR HEALTH AND WEIGHT LOSS

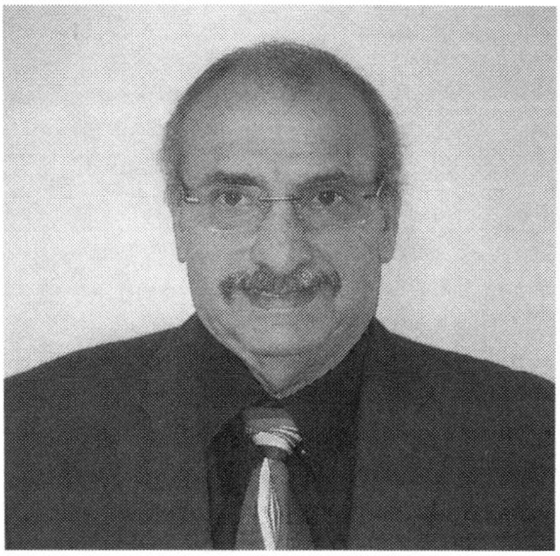

Dr. Hashem Fehmi Yasin

Publisher: For bulk sales and permissions.
Dr. Hashem Fehmi Yasin
34650 Cowan Road
Westland, Michigan 48185-7121
Phone: (313) 284-5949
Fax: 734-396-1066
Email: drhashemfyasin@gmail.com
ISBN:

Dedications:

For Mom, Mercedes Cerón de Yasin.
To my beloved mother, 86 years old, whom I love deeply. Thank you for your unconditional love and for every one of your good deeds, which have been a beacon of light for all your children. For years we practiced intermittent fasting and the ketogenic diet together to improve our health. This book is for you.

And

For Iris Jiménez Yasin, my beloved wife.
Thank you for your companionship, your unconditional support, and for sharing with me this journey of intermittent fasting and the ketogenic diet. This book is a token of my love and gratitude toward you.

Acknowledgments:

I want to express my deepest gratitude to all the people who made the creation of this book possible.

To my wife, Iris Jiménez Yasin, for her invaluable support, patience, and for being the tireless editor who gave shape to my ideas. Her dedication and love are the force behind every word.

To my dear mother, Mercedes Cerón de Yasin, for being the constant inspiration in my life and for teaching me the value of effort and perseverance.

To my children and all my family, whose love and encouragement have driven me to move forward with this project.

To my friends and colleagues, for their valuable feedback and for their belief in my work.

Finally, to every reader. I hope this book provides you with valuable knowledge and inspires you on your own journey toward a healthier life.

Table Of Contents

Chapter 8: Beyond Weight Loss: Health Benefits of Fasting and Keto

- Exploring the broader health implications (reduced risk of chronic diseases, improved insulin sensitivity).
- Discussing mental health benefits.
- Testimonials from individuals who have experienced holistic improvements.

Chapter 9: Lifestyle Integration

- Tips on how to incorporate intermittent keto fasting into a busy lifestyle.
- Social considerations (eating out, holidays, and special occasions).
- Maintaining a balance without feelings of deprivation.

Conclusion

- Recap the main points discussed in the book.
- Encourage readers to experiment and find the right balance for their bodies.
- Inspire ongoing learning and adaptation in their health journey.

Key Themes and Messages

Simplicity and Accessibility: Emphasize that intermittent fasting and the ketogenic diet can be easily integrated into daily life with some planning.

- Empowerment through Knowledge: Provide readers with the scientific basis to help them make informed decisions regarding their health.
- Sustainability: Highlight that this approach is not just a quick fix, but a sustainable way to improve health and well-being.
- FAQ Section: Address common questions and concerns about intermittent fasting and keto.
- Bonus Chapter: Exercise and how it complements intermittent fasting and keto for maximum health benefits.

Additional Elements

- Appendices: Glossary of terms,
- additional reading materials,
- links to online communities.

Introduction: A New Path to Good Health

For many people, the journey to a healthier life can feel like a myriad of conflicting advice and complicated rules. You're told to count every calorie, restrict lots of food groups, or spend hours at the gym. It's easy to feel overwhelmed and, over time, lose motivation. What if there was a different way? A path that isn't about deprivation but a more innovative, more sustainable approach to your body's natural processes.

Welcome to a new way of thinking about your health, combining two potent dietary strategies today: **Intermittent Fasting (IF)** and the **Ketogenic (Keto) Diet**. You may have heard of them individually. Intermittent fasting is a way of eating with periods of eating and fasting, without focusing on what you eat, but rather *when* you eat. On the other hand, the ketogenic diet is all about what you eat—a high-fat, very low-carbohydrate approach designed to shift your body's metabolism from burning sugar to burning fat for fuel.

This book is a guide to combining these two powerful methods. We'll show you how they work together to make a powerful synergy that can accelerate weight loss, improve metabolic health, and offer many other benefits far beyond the scale. We'll strip away the complexity and provide a clear, practical road map so you can feel empowered to take control of your health. This isn't about a quick fix or another short-lived diet; it's about giving you the knowledge and helping you make lasting changes that fit into your daily life.

By the end of this book, you won't just know what to do; you'll understand *why* it works. You'll have the tools to unlock your body's potential for sustainable health and well-being.

Preface

The traditional approach to health and weight loss—based on counting calories and restricting foods—often leads to frustration and failure. This method ignores the body's hormonal and metabolic environment, creating a cycle of insulin spikes that promotes fat storage.

This book proposes a new way of thinking, combining Intermittent Fasting (IF) and the Ketogenic Diet (Keto) to create a powerful synergy. Unlike conventional diets, this approach is not about deprivation, but about working with your body's innate intelligence.

- **Intermittent Fasting (IF):** Focuses on *when* you eat. During fasting periods, insulin levels drop, allowing the body to burn fat and activate autophagy, a cellular cleansing process. Fasting also improves brain function and mental clarity.

- **Ketogenic Diet (Keto):** Focuses on *what* you eat. By drastically reducing carbohydrates, the body enters ketosis—a state in which it burns fat for energy in the form of ketones. This provides steady energy, eliminates cravings, and reduces inflammation.

- **Together, IF and Keto complement each other perfectly.** The keto diet prepares the body to burn fat, making fasting easier and more efficient. In turn, fasting helps achieve a deeper state of ketosis. This combination simplifies the process, as you'll have a clear framework of what to eat (Keto) and when to eat (IF), freeing you from the need to count calories.

In short, this book is a practical guide for lasting lifestyle change, designed to help you regain your energy, improve your metabolic health, and take control of your well-being in a sustainable and empowering way.

Chapter 1: Understanding Intermittent Fasting

Before we discuss combining intermittent fasting with the ketogenic diet, we must understand each of them separately. Let's begin with a closer look at intermittent fasting.

At its core, **intermittent fasting (IF)** is not a diet but an eating pattern. It's a structured approach that cycles between eating and voluntary fasting periods. The key idea isn't *what* you eat but *when* you eat. This simple shift in timing allows your body to tap into its natural metabolic processes, which can lead to significant health benefits.

Popular Methods of Intermittent Fasting

There's no single way to do intermittent fasting. The most effective method is often the one you can stick with long-term. Here are three of the most popular approaches:

- **The 16/8 Method:** This is arguably the most common and beginner-friendly method. It is fasting for 16 hours and eating all your meals in an 8-hour window. For example, you might eat between 12:00 PM. and 8:00 PM., then fast for the rest of the day and night. This method is popular because it often just means skipping breakfast and having your first meal at lunchtime.
- **The 5:2 Method:** With this approach, you eat normally five days a week. On the other two days, you significantly restrict your calorie intake, typically 500-600 calories. These "fasting days" are non-consecutive, giving you a balance throughout the week.
- **The Eat-Stop-Eat Method** involves a 24-hour fast, once or twice a week. A person might eat dinner on Monday, then not eat again until dinner on Tuesday. This is a more advanced method and can take some getting used to.

- **The Science Behind the Fast**

Why does simply changing your eating schedule work so well? The benefits of intermittent fasting stem from several key biological changes that happen in your body during a fasted state:

- **Insulin Sensitivity and levels in blood:** After eating, your body raises insulin to help your cells absorb the new glucose from your blood. When you're constantly eating, your insulin levels stay high, and your cells can become resistant to the effects. Fasting gives your body a break, allowing insulin levels to drop and your cells to become more sensitive again. This is crucial for weight management and preventing chronic diseases that are becoming part of our lives.
- **Hormonal Boosts:** Your body's **Human Growth Hormone (HGH)** levels increase dramatically during a fast. HGH is vital for muscle growth, fat loss, and overall vitality. Fasting also increases norepinephrine, which signals fat cells to break down body fat into energy.
- **Cellular Repair or Autophagy:** Fasting starts a process called autophagy, which is self-eating. This is your body's way of cleaning the house. It removes damaged cells and reuses the components. Autophagy is a powerful mechanism for cellular renewal and has been linked to longevity and disease prevention.

Intermittent fasting allows these beneficial processes to kick in by allowing your body to rest from digestion. This will help you lose weight, improve your metabolic health, and feel more energized.

Chapter 2: The Ketogenic Diet Explained

Now that you understand intermittent fasting, let's focus on the second half of this powerful duo: the ketogenic diet. While intermittent fasting dictates *when* you eat, the ketogenic diet defines *what* you eat, creating a metabolic state that is incredibly effective for health and weight management.

What is a Ketogenic Diet?

The ketogenic diet, or "keto" for short, is a very low-carbohydrate, high-fat, and moderate-protein eating plan. The goal is to reduce your carb intake and replace it with fat dramatically. This shift forces your body into a metabolic state called **ketosis**.

In a normal state, your body's primary fuel source is glucose, which comes from carbohydrates. When you restrict carbs, your body has to find an alternative fuel. Then, your liver begins to break down fat cells into molecules called **ketones**, which become the new primary fuel source for your body and brain. Our ancestors relied on this natural metabolic process when food was scarce.

Key Benefits of the Ketogenic Diet

The switch to using ketones for fuel has a wide range of benefits that go beyond simple weight loss:

- **Accelerated Fat Loss:** By definition, a ketogenic diet trains your body to become a "fat-burning machine." When you're in ketosis, you're constantly tapping into your fat stores for energy, leading to efficient and often rapid weight loss.
- **Improved Metabolic Health:** A keto diet can significantly improve insulin sensitivity, which regulates blood sugar levels and can be particularly beneficial for those with pre-diabetes or type 2 diabetes. Lowered insulin levels also make accessing and burning stored fat easier for the body.

- **Enhanced Brain Function:** Your brain can run on either glucose or ketones. Most people report improved mental clarity, focus, and reduced "brain fog" when in ketosis. Ketones are a clean and efficient fuel source for the brain, and the diet may have neuroprotective effects.

Common Misconceptions

There are a few myths about the ketogenic diet that are important to clear up:

- **"Keto is just about eating bacon and butter."** While the diet is high in fat, the quality of that fat is crucial. The best ketogenic diets are rich in many healthy fats from sources like avocados, olive oil, nuts, and fatty fish, alongside a generous intake of non-starchy vegetables.
- **"Keto is dangerous."** For most healthy individuals, a well-formulated ketogenic diet is safe. The "keto flu," a temporary period of fatigue and headaches, can occur as your body transitions to ketosis, but it's typically a short-lived adjustment period.
- **"You can't eat vegetables."** On the contrary, leafy greens and other low-carb vegetables are essential for providing fiber, vitamins, and minerals vital for overall health.

The ketogenic diet is a powerful way to transform health by focusing on whole, nutrient-dense foods.

Chapter 3: The Synergy of Intermittent Fasting and Keto methods

You've now learned about intermittent fasting, a powerful tool for timing your meals, and the ketogenic diet, a metabolic strategy for fueling your body with fat. On their own, each is a remarkable approach to health. But when combined, they create a far more powerful synergy than the sum of their parts. This is where the magic truly happens.

Fasting: The Express Lane to Ketosis

Think of your body's energy system as having two primary modes: sugar-burning and fat-burning modes. Your body prefers to use sugar (glucose) first. You must deplete your body's glycogen (stored glucose) reserves to get into ketosis. This can take a few days on a standard keto diet.

This is where intermittent fasting provides a considerable advantage. Extending the period between meals, you naturally deplete your glycogen stores much faster. For instance, a 16-hour fast can significantly reduce your liver's glycogen, paving a smoother and quicker path into ketosis. You're not just restricting carbs; you're also giving your body an extended period to burn through its existing fuel source, making the metabolic transition to burning fat for fuel easier and more efficient. This reduces the time it takes to enter ketosis and can help mitigate the dreaded "keto flu."

Amplified Benefits and Research-Backed Results

While research on the combined approach is still emerging, studies have indicated that combining intermittent fasting and keto can lead to several amplified benefits:

- **Increased Fat Burning:** The low insulin levels from a keto diet and the hormonal changes triggered by fasting (like increased norepinephrine) create an optimal environment for your body to access and burn stubborn fat stores.

- **Enhanced Autophagy:** The cellular cleanup process of autophagy, a key benefit of fasting, is often enhanced when the body is in a state of ketosis, a stress-resistant metabolic state. This can lead to greater cellular renewal and anti-aging benefits.
- **Improved Brain Health:** When your brain runs on ketones, it has a steady and sure clean alternative fuel, along with the cellular repair of fasting, it may give enhanced mental protection and clarity.

Real Life Success Story

For many, combining these two methods is a game-changer. These aren't just stories of weight loss, but of holistic transformation:

- A busy parent who struggled with evening snacking found that the 16/8 fasting schedule and satisfying keto meals eliminated cravings and led to a consistent 20-pound weight loss.
- A fitness enthusiast who had hit a weight-loss plateau discovered that adding a weekly 24-hour fast to their keto routine helped them break through and achieve a new body composition and energy level.
- Professionals who felt constantly tired and "foggy" found that the intermittent keto approach's mental clarity and sustained energy transformed their productivity and well-being, proving it wasn't just about the scale.

The power of this combination is in its elegant simplicity: it works with your body's natural processes, not against them. In the next chapter, we'll view the "why" and the "how," providing you with the practical steps to start your own journey.

Chapter 4: Getting Started

You know—now it's time to put it into action. Beginning a new lifestyle can feel daunting, but remember that this is a journey, not a race. The key is to start slow, be consistent, and listen to your body. This chapter will provide the essential tools and practical tips to transition into the intermittent keto lifestyle successfully.

Practical Tips for Beginning Your Journey

- **Start with Keto First:** For many people, it's easier to first adapt to the ketogenic diet for a week or two before introducing a strict fasting schedule. This allows your body to become "fat-adapted" and reduces the initial shock of changing both *what* you eat and *when* you eat.
- **Stay Hydrated and Electrolytes are Key:** As you transition into ketosis, your body will lose water and essential minerals. To prevent the "keto flu," drinking plenty of water and replenishing your electrolytes is crucial. And adding a pinch of salt to your water, and consider supplements for magnesium and potassium if needed.
- **Prioritize Sleep:** Sleep is one of the most powerful tools for managing your metabolism and hormones. The aim is for 7-9 hours of quality sleep each night. This will help reduce cravings, manage cortisol levels, and support your body's adaptation process.
- **Listen to Your Body:** Pay attention to how you feel. While some hunger is normal during a fast, you should never feel deprived or sick. If you're struggling with a 16-hour fast, try a 12-hour fast first and gradually increase the duration. There is no one-size-fits-all approach.

Transitioning and Finding Your Fasting Schedule

Your first step is to choose a simple fasting schedule. The **16/8 method** is an excellent starting point.

- **Choose your 8-hour eating window:** A popular choice is 12:00 PM to 8:00 PM. This means you'll skip breakfast, have your first meal by noon, and finish your last meal by 8 PM.
- **Ease into it:** If skipping breakfast feels too difficult, start by delaying it by just an hour or two. Gradually push back your first meal until you comfortably reach the 16-hour fasting window.
- **Stay busy:** Distractions are your friend during the fasting window. Drink black coffee, green tea, or water. Go for a walk, work on a project, or read a book. The time will fly by.

Sample Grocery List and Meal Prep Ideas

Having the right foods on hand is essential to make this joyful journey simple. This is a basic grocery list you need to start:

Proteins:

- Beef, chicken, pork
- Salmon, tuna, and other fatty fish
- Eggs

Healthy Fats:

- Avocados and avocado oil
- Olive oil
- Nuts (almonds, macadamia nuts) and seeds (chia, flax)
- Butter, ghee, coconut oil

Low-Carb Vegetables:

- Leafy greens (spinach, kale, lettuce)
- Broccoli, cauliflower, asparagus
- Bell peppers, zucchini, cucumbers

Dairy (in moderation):

- Hard cheeses
- Heavy cream
- Full-fat Greek yogurt (check for low-carb varieties)

Meal Prep Ideas:

- **Make a batch of protein:** Cook a whole chicken or a significant portion of ground beef. This can be used for salads, wraps (using lettuce), or as a side for quick meals.
- **Chop vegetables:** Pre-chop your broccoli, bell peppers, and other low-carb vegetables so they are ready to use for stir-fries or salads.
- **Prepare a fatty dressing:** Make a simple vinaigrette with olive oil, vinegar, and herbs. This can be used for multiple meals throughout the week.

By preparing ahead of time, you remove the stress of figuring out what to eat each day and set yourself up for success.

Chapter 5: Meal Planning for Success

With your pantry stocked and your fasting schedule in mind, the next step is to plan your meals. Meal planning is one of the most powerful tools for staying on track with intermittent fasting and the ketogenic diet. It removes the stress of daily decision-making, prevents impulsive eating, and ensures you're consistently fueling your body with the right nutrients.

Sample Meal Plans

Here are two sample meal plans designed to give you a clear idea of what a day of eating might look like on an intermittent keto schedule.

Sample Plan: 16/8 Fast

- **Fast from** 8:00 PM. to 12:00 PM. the next day.
- **Meal 1 (12:00 PM):** A large, nutrient-dense salad with mixed greens, grilled chicken or salmon, avocado, nuts, and a creamy olive oil-based dressing.
- **Snack (3:00 PM):** A handful of almonds, macadamia nuts, or a small piece of cheese.
- **Meal 2 (7:00 PM):** Sheet-pan roasted sausage and bell peppers with steamed broccoli.

Sample Plan: 24-Hour Fast (Eat-Stop-Eat)

- **Last Meal (Monday 7:00 PM):** A hearty keto chili with ground beef, cheese, and sour cream.
- **Fast from** 7:00 PM Monday to 7:00 PM Tuesday. Only drink unsweetened water, black coffee, or tea during this time.
- **First Meal (Tuesday 7:00 PM):** A filling, celebratory keto meal like a grass-fed steak with a generous portion of asparagus sauteed in butter.

Easy Keto-Friendly Recipes

You don’t need to be a chef to eat well on a ketogenic diet. Here are a few simple recipes perfect for meal prepping and daily meals.

Quick & Easy Keto Salad

- **Ingredients:** 2 cups of mixed greens, ½ cup of cooked and cooled shredded chicken, ¼ cup of sliced avocado, 2 tbsps of feta cheese, 2 tbsps of toasted pumpkin seeds, and a dressing made from 3 tbsps of olive oil, 1 tbsp of apple cider vinegar, salt, and pepper.
- **Instructions:** Combine all ingredients in a bowl. Toss with the dressing just before serving.

Fat-Fueled Smoothie

- **Ingredients are:** 1 cup of unsweetened almond milk, ½ cup of spinach, 1 scoop of low-carb protein powder, 1 tbsp of almond butter, and ice.
- **Instructions:** Blend all ingredients until smooth. This is a great, quick meal replacement that's especially useful for a post-fast meal.

Simple Sheet Pan Chicken & Veggies

- **Ingredients:** 2 lbs of chicken thighs, one large head of broccoli, one red bell pepper, one zucchini, 3 tbsp of avocado oil, salt, pepper, and garlic powder.
- **Instruction:** Heat the oven to 400°F (200°C); toss the chicken and chopped vegetables with avocado oil and seasonings on a large baking sheet. Roast for 20-25 minutes, or til the chicken is cooked through and the vegetables are tender.

Balanced Meals to get Optimal Nutrition

When you plan your meals, it's important to ensure you're ingesting various nutrients, even with a low-carb intake. A good rule of thumb for every meal is to build your plate around these three components:

1. **A source of high-quality protein** is vital for muscle maintenance and satiety. Think chicken, fish, eggs, or beef.
2. **A generous portion of healthy fats:** These fuel your body on a keto diet and help you feel full and satisfied. Include avocados, olive oil, nuts, or fatty fish.
3. **Plenty of low-carb vegetables** provide essential vitamins, minerals, and fiber. Mix half your plate with non-starchy veggies like leafy greens, broccoli, and cauliflower.

Focusing on these building blocks allows you to easily create balanced, delicious, and satisfying meals without feeling restricted.

Ready to tackle some of the common hurdles you might face? Let's move on to Chapter 6: Common Challenges and Solutions.

Chapter 6: Common Challenges and Solutions

Embarking on any new health journey comes with its own set of challenges. It's completely normal to face a few bumps in the road, especially in the beginning. Being prepared for these common issues and knowing how to handle them is a crucial part of long-term success. This chapter will provide practical solutions to the most frequent obstacles you might encounter.

Addressing the Keto Flu and Gastric Issues

As your body changes from burning carbs to burning fat fuel, you may experience a temporary period of fatigue, headaches, or irritability known as the "keto flu." This is not a sign that something is wrong; it's simply your body adapting to a new metabolic state.

Solutions:

- **Hydrate Aggressively:** Drink more water than you think you need. Staying well-hydrated is the number one defense against keto flu symptoms.
- **Replenish Electrolytes:** Your body flushes out sodium, potassium, and magnesium as it sheds water weight. This mineral loss is a primary cause of keto flu. You can combat this by adding one gram of sea salt to your water or broth, eating foods high in potassium like avocados, and taking a magnesium pill.
- **Ease into it:** If symptoms are severe, consider a more gradual reduction of carbs. Slowing down and having your body adapt at its own pace is okay.

Digestive issues, such as constipation, can also happen when you first start. This is often due to lack of fiber.

Solutions:

- **Eat Your Vegetables:** Ensure your meals are rich in low-carb, high-fiber vegetables like leafy greens, broccoli, and cauliflower.
- **Stay Hydrated:** Drinking 2 liters of water is essential to keep things moving in your digestive tract.

Overcoming Hunger Pangs While Fasting

Your mind and body are used to a specific eating way, so it's natural to feel hunger pangs at first. The good news is that these pangs often come in waves and will eventually pass.

Solutions:

- **Drink, Drink, Drink:** When hunger strikes, have a large glass of water, a cup of black coffee, or some herbal tea. These can help curb your appetite and fill your stomach.
- **Distract Yourself:** Use the time you would typically spend eating to focus on a task, go for a walk, or read a book. Keeping your mind busy can make the fasting window fly by.
- **Fuel Your Body Right:** Ensure your eating window meals are full of satisfying, healthy fats and protein. A well-formulated keto meal will keep you satiated for much longer than a carb-heavy one.

Staying Motivated and Accountable

Motivation can be low and flow when it feels challenging to stick with the plan; having a system in place can make all the difference.

Solutions are:

- **Remember Your Reasons "Why":** Connect with the core reason you started this journey. Is it for more energy? To be more present with your family? To improve your health? Remind yourself of this goal often.
- **Find a Support System:** Share your journey with a friend, join an online community, or work with a coach. Having others to share your successes and challenges can make a huge difference.
- **Track Your Progress:** Keep a journal of your weight, energy levels, mood, sleep quality, and how your clothes fit. These non-scale victories are powerful boosters.

By treating these challenges as standard parts of the process, you can navigate them with confidence and stay on your path to better health.

Chapter 7: Monitoring Progress and Making the Adjustments

You've begun your journey, faced the initial challenges, and are now moving forward. But how do you know if what you're doing is actually working? While the number on the scale is one metric, it's far from the only one. A combination of factors measures true success. This chapter will provide the tools to track your progress and the knowledge to adjust your strategy when needed.

Tools and Techniques for Tracking Progress

To get a comprehensive picture of your progress, it's essential to look beyond your weight.

- **Non-Scale Victories (NSVs):** These are often the most powerful indicators of success. Pay attention to how your clothes fit, the increase in your energy levels, improved mental clarity, better sleep, and a more stable mood, and take a moment each week to reflect on these changes and celebrate them.
- **Body Measurement:** Use a tape measure to track areas like your waist, hips, and thighs. Weight fluctuations are normal, but a consistent decrease in these measurements is a clear sign of fat loss.
- **Progress Photos:** While it might feel uncomfortable at first, taking weekly or bi-weekly photos of yourself from the front, side, and back is an incredibly motivating way to see gradual change.
- **Journaling:** Record how you feel daily, what you eat, and your fasting. It is to help you identify patterns and understand what works best for your body.

When to Adjust Your Strategy

The intermittent keto approach is not a rigid plan, but a flexible framework. You are the expert on your own body, and knowing when to adjust is a sign of empowerment.

- **If you hit a plateau:** If you've been consistent for a few weeks but the scale or your measurements haven't budged, it might be time to make a small change. Try shortening or lengthening your eating window, or slightly adjusting your macro amounts.
- **If you're feeling bad:** You are feeling lethargic, overly hungry, or irritable after initially adapting, it may be a sign that your fasting schedule or your macro breakdown isn't right for you. It's okay to scale back to a more comfortable fasting window or re-evaluate your food choices.
- **If you want to intensify your efforts:** Once you are comfortable with your current regimen, try a longer fast (like a weekly 24-hour fast) or be more disciplined with your macro tracking to see if that yields new results.

The key is to make one change at a time, track the results for a week or two, and then decide if it's working.

Maintaining Long-Term Success

This is not a temporary solution; it's about building a sustainable lifestyle.

- **Flexibility is key:** Don't let a single "off-plan" meal or day derail you. One meal doesn't erase your progress. Acknowledge it and get right back on track with your next meal or fast.
- **Focus on habits, not willpower:** Make the routines easy to follow. Meal prep, for instance, makes a huge difference. The less you rely on willpower, the more likely you are to stick with it.

- **Embrace the journey:** See this as a lifelong exploration of your health, not a destination. As your body changes, your needs may change too. Stay curious, stay informed, and always listen to the signals your body is giving you.

By tracking your progress and confidently making the changes, you can make sure that your journey will be effective, enjoyable, and sustainable for the long haul.

Chapter 8: More than Weight Loss: The Benefits of Fasting Keto

Your diet may have started with a goal to lose weight, but the benefits of combining intermittent fasting and the ketogenic diet extend far beyond the number of pounds lost. This lifestyle is a powerful tool for overall health and well-being, influencing everything from your metabolism to your mental clarity. This chapter will explore the profound, holistic improvements you can expect.

The Broader Health Implications

Weight loss is a positive side effect of a good metabolic shift. By prioritizing whole foods and giving your body a break from constant digestion, you're creating an internal environment that is primed for good health.

- **Improved Insulin Sensitivity:** The constant intake of carbohydrates, such as sugars and flours, leads to insulin resistance, type 2 diabetes, and other chronic diseases. Both fasting and a low-carb diet work to lower insulin levels. When combined, this effect is amplified, helping your body become more sensitive to insulin. This not only aids in weight loss but is a crucial step in disease prevention.
- **Reduced Inflammation:** Chronic, low-grade inflammation is now understood to be a major factor in many modern diseases. Research suggests that both fasting and a ketogenic diet can have powerful anti-inflammatory effects. By reducing the load of inflammatory foods and giving your body time to reset, you are helping to calm this systemic inflammation.
- **Cardiovascular Health:** The intermittent keto approach can improve key markers of heart health, with a marked reduction in triglycerides and an increase in HDL (good) cholesterol.

The Mental Health and Cognitive Benefit

The physical benefit is significant, but many people report that the mental and cognitive improvement is what truly makes this lifestyle sustainable.

- **Enhanced Mental Clarity:** When your brain is fueled by ketones, you get a clean, steady source of energy. This can lead to a significant reduction in brain fog and a newfound sense of mental clarity and focus. The roller coaster of highs and lows in blood sugar is eliminated, giving you stable energy throughout the day.
- **Improved Mood and Stability:** The consistent energy supply to the brain, combined with the reduction in inflammation, can have a stabilizing effect on mood. Many people report feeling more balanced, less anxious, and more confident in their daily lives.

Holistic Improvements: Testimonial

These health changes often lead to a renewed sense of confidence and high feeling of well-being. Here are just a few examples of the holistic transformations people have experienced:

- "I started this to lose 15 pounds, but the biggest change wasn't the number on the scale. It was the energy I have now to play with my kids and the mental focus I have at work. I feel like I got my vitality back."
- "My cravings for sugar are completely gone. The confidence I've gained from knowing I can control what I eat, rather than food controlling me, is a game-changer. I am a completely different person."
- "After years of feeling sluggish and 'off,' the combination of fasting and keto helped me regain a sense of control over my

health. I not only lost weight, but I also slept better, and my doctor says my blood work has never looked better."

The true reward of this lifestyle is not just looking better, but feeling better—empowered, healthy, and in tune with your body's needs.

Chapter 9: Lifestyle Integration

The successful health journey isn't just about what you do at home, but it's about how you integrate those habits into the world. A sustainable lifestyle must be easy enough to handle busy schedules, social events, and special occasions without causing stress or guilt. This chapter will provide you with the tools to make intermittent keto a natural, effortless part of your life.

Tips for a Busy Lifestyle

- **Plan Ahead:** Take 15 minutes at the beginning of the week to map out your meals and fasting windows. This simple act of planning can keep you from impulsive eating on a hectic day.
- **Meal Prep Strategically:** Cook large batches of protein (like chicken or ground beef) and chop vegetables on Sunday. This gives you easy, ready-to-go options for your meals during the week, especially on days when you have no time to cook.
- **Be Flexible with Your Fasting:** Your fasting window doesn't have to be the exact same time every day. On a day with an early dinner, you might start your fast a little earlier. If you have a late lunch planned, you can simply push back your first meal. The key is to find a rhythm that works for you, not the other way around.

Navigating Social Occasions and Holidays

The fear of social isolation is a major reason many people abandon a new way of eating. With the right mindset and a few simple, well-planned strategies, you can enjoy these moments without derailing your progress.

- **Eating Out:** Don't be afraid to look at the menu online before you go. Most restaurants offer keto-friendly options like grilled meats, salads with full-fat dressings, and bunless burgers. You can also ask for simple substitutions, such as swapping out a side of potatoes for steamed vegetables.

- **Holidays and Celebrations:** It's okay to indulge strategically. If there is a special meal you want to enjoy, have it without guilt and regrets. The beauty of this lifestyle is the flexibility. Just one single meal will not erase weeks of good habits attained. on the next day, simply get back on track with your fasting and keto eating. It's a marathon, not a sprint, and these moments are what make life rich.

Maintaining Balance Without Deprivation

The feeling of deprivation is the enemy of sustainability. When you feel like you're missing out, it becomes a mental battle that is difficult to win long-term.

- **Focus on What You Can Eat:** The world of keto is full of delicious and satisfying foods. Instead of mourning the absence of bread and pasta, fall in love with creamy avocados, rich cheeses, savory roasted meats, and flavorful, crisp vegetables.
- **Enjoy the Simplicity:** There is a freedom in not having to constantly decide what to eat. The structure of intermittent fasting and the clarity of the keto diet can simplify your life and reduce decision fatigue, leaving you with more energy for the things that really matter.
- **Build a Foundation of Health and Progress:** When you focus on the long-term benefits of sustained energy, mental clarity, and overall well-being, the cravings for quick-fix junk food will naturally diminish. You're not giving anything up; you're simply choosing better for yourself.

Making this a sustainable way of life is a practice of awareness, flexibility, and compassion for yourself. It is about finding a lifestyle that feels great and works with your life, not against it.

Conclusion: A Sustainable Journey to the Optimal Health you will get

You now reached the end of this guide. But now, the real journey is just beginning. You've been equipped with a new understanding of your body, a powerful set of tools, and a practical road map to a healthy life.

We have covered the fundamentals of **intermittent fasting** and learned that timing your meals can unlock your body's natural fat-burning and repair mechanisms. You've also discovered the metabolic power of the **ketogenic diet**, which shifts your body from a sugar-dependent state to a fat-fueled machine. Most importantly, you now know how these two approaches work in perfect **synergy**, creating an amplified effect that leads to more efficient weight loss and a host of other health benefits.

This book has shown you how to move from theory to practice—how to get started, plan your meals for success, and overcome common challenges. You've learned to focus on **non-scale victories** and listen to the signals your body is sending you, empowering you to make adjustments and take control of your own health narrative.

The goal of this lifestyle is not just to lose a specific number of pounds on the scale, but to achieve a profound and lasting feeling of well-being. It is about having more energy, experiencing more mental clarity, and feeling confident in your manner to nourish and care for yourself. It is a path of **empowerment through knowledge** and **sustainability through simplicity**.

As you move forward, remember to be patient and compassionate with yourself. This is not perfection, but it is progress. Join the flexibility of this way of life and trust in the process. You have all the tools you need to build a healthier, more vibrant life.

FAQ: Your Quick Guide to Common Questions

Even with a detailed plan, questions will inevitably come up. This section provides quick, clear answers to the most frequent concerns about combining intermittent fasting and the ketogenic diet.

Can I exercise while fasting?

Yes, absolutely. Many people find that they have more energy for exercise, especially low-to-moderate intensity workouts, during a fasted state. Fasting may even enhance the fat-burning effects of your workout. If you are doing an intense workout, a pre-workout snack (like a bulletproof coffee) may be beneficial, or you can schedule your workout at the beginning of your eating window.

What can I drink during my fasting window?

During your fasting window, stick to beverages that won't break your fast. These include:

- **Water** (still or sparkling)
- **Black coffee** (without cream, sugar, or sweeteners)
- **Plain green or black tea**
- **Herbal tea**

These beverages have virtually no calories and will not trigger an insulin response.

What if I get hungry during a fast?

Hunger pangs are normal, especially at the beginning, but they often come in waves. The best strategies are to:

- **Drink large glasses of water, coffee, or tea.**

- **Stay busy** to distract yourself.
- **Remember your "why"**—your long-term health goals.

As your body adapts to fat for fuel, you'll likely find that hunger becomes much easier to manage.

What if I have a "cheat" meal?

A single high-carb meal will temporarily take you out of ketosis, but it will not erase your progress. The key is to get right back on track with your next meal or fast. Think of it as a temporary halt, not the end of your journey. The intermittent keto lifestyle is about consistency.

Will I lose muscle mass while fasting?

This is a common concern. Research suggests that intermittent fasting, especially when combined with adequate protein intake and strength training during the eating window, does not lead to a significant loss of muscle mass. In fact, the boost in Human Growth Hormone (HGH) that occurs during a fast can help with muscle preservation.

Do I need to take supplements?

The most important supplements, especially at the beginning, are **electrolytes** (sodium, potassium, and magnesium) to help with keto flu symptoms. A good-quality multivitamin can also help fill in any nutritional gaps. Consult with your doctor or dietitian before using any new vitamins or supplements.

Bonus Chapter: Exercise, the Final Catalyst

You now have a powerful understanding of how to use intermittent fasting and the ketogenic diet to transform your health from the inside out. But to truly unlock your body's full potential, there is one more key element: exercise. When combined with your new lifestyle, physical activity acts as a powerful catalyst, accelerating your results and reinforcing all the benefits you've learned about.

The Synergy of Movement and Metabolism

Exercise and the intermittent keto approach work in a virtuous cycle. When you do physical activity, you will burn more calories and deplete your glycogen stores, which helps you enter ketosis faster and more efficiently. At the same time, being in a state of ketosis gives your body a sustained, clean fuel source for your workouts, meaning you can often exercise with more energy and stamina than on a carb-heavy diet.

This combination also amplifies the hormonal benefits. The increase in Human Growth Hormone (HGH) from fasting, combined with a workout, is a powerful recipe for muscle preservation and fat burning. You teach your body to become a highly efficient, fat-burning machine.

Choosing the Right Workout for Your Lifestyle

The best exercise is the one you enjoy and will keep doing. Consider these guidelines for introducing different types of workouts into your routine:

Low-to-Moderate Intensity Exercise (Fasted State)

Exercises like walking, jogging, hiking, cycling, and yoga are excellent choices for a fasted state. They are primarily fueled by fat, so your body is perfectly primed for them. A morning walk or a light workout before your first meal can be a great way to start your day, burn some extra fat, and get a boost of mental clarity.

High-Intensity & Strength Training (Fed State)

For workouts that require explosive power, like weightlifting, High-Intensity Interval Training (HIIT), or sprints, you may benefit from having some fuel in your system. This doesn't mean you need a carb-heavy meal; a small, keto-friendly snack like a handful of nuts or protein powder can provide the quick energy your muscles need. It's often best to schedule these workouts at the start of your eating window to replenish your energy with your first meal.

Key Tips for Success

- **Stay Hydrated:** Drink at least 2 liters of water before, during, and after your workout, especially if you're exercising while fasted.
- **Listen to Your Body:** Pay attention to how you feel. If a fasted workout makes you feel light-headed or unwell, it's okay to try it after your first meal instead.
- **Consistency over Intensity:** It's far better to do a moderate workout three to four times a week than one or two intense sessions you can't sustain.

By adding a regular exercise routine to your intermittent keto lifestyle, you are not only accelerating your results but also building a more substantial, more resilient body. This is the final step in creating a complete, holistic strategy for your long-term health and well-being.

Appendix A: Glossary of Terms

Here are some of the key terms you encountered in this book, defined simply to help you on your journey.

- **Intermittent Fasting (IF):** Is a way of eating and fasting cycles, periods of not eating or voluntary fasting. It focuses on *when* you eat, rather than *what* you eat.
- **Ketogenic Diet (Keto):** A high-fat, moderate-protein, and very low-carbohydrate eating plan designed to shift the body's metabolism into a state of ketosis.
- **Ketosis:** A natural metabolic state where your body primarily burns fat for fuel, producing molecules called ketones for energy.
- **Ketones:** Molecules produced in the liver from fat when carbohydrate intake is very low. They are an alternative fuel source for the body and brain.

- **Macronutrients:** The three main components of food that the body needs for energy: carbohydrates, fats, and proteins.
- **Autophagy:** A cellular "self-cleaning" process that is triggered during fasting. It helps the body remove and recycle old, damaged cells.
- **Electrolytes:** Essential minerals like sodium, potassium, and magnesium that the body needs to function correctly. They are crucial for preventing the "keto flu."
- **Keto Flu:** A temporary period of side effects—such as fatigue, headaches, or irritability—that can occur as your body changes from burning sugar to burning ketones or fat shows good adaptation.

Appendix B: Further Resources

This is not an exhaustive list, but a starting point for further learning and community support.

Online Communities

Connecting with others on the same purpose can be a powerful source of motivation and practical advice. Looking for forums or social media groups dedicated to intermittent fasting, the ketogenic diet, or both. These communities often share recipes, success stories, and encouragement.

Additional Reading

Look for books and articles from doctors, nutritionists, and researchers specializing in these topics. Seeking information from multiple reputable sources will help you deepen your understanding and find new strategies.

About the Author: Hashem Fehmi Yasin

Hashem Fehmi Yasin is a multifaceted professional with vast experience in the legal, medical, and business fields. With a solid academic background in law, dentistry, and medicine—complemented by his fluency in Spanish, English, and Arabic—his career is a testament to his versatility and adaptability.

From his beginnings as General Manager at Matta's Fine Foods and owner of Five Golden Stars, Hashem has demonstrated sharp business acumen. His professional path evolved to include roles such as Legal Associate at Yasin Enterprises International in the Dominican Republic and, notably, as a Professor of Medicine at Universidad Federico Henríquez y Carvajal.

His commitment to service and communication is reflected in his work as an interpreter and translator for the US Federal and State Courts, a role he has carried out since 2011. He is currently the CEO of Legal Inc. and a notary public in Michigan.

In addition to his impressive professional record, Hashem is a commercial pilot and has a strong interest in computing and aviation. His dedication to lifelong learning and his rich life experience provide him with a unique and profound perspective, making him an author with a truly global and diverse vision.

Dr. Hashem Fehmi Yasin is also a researcher and healthcare professional passionate about the study of human nutrition and metabolism. Throughout his career, he has devoted his work to integrating science, clinical experience, and modern strategies to help people achieve a healthier lifestyle.

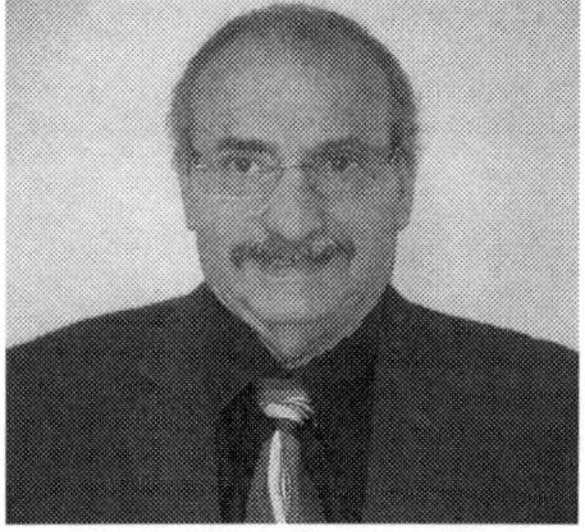

Made in the USA
Monee, IL
04 November 2026

67384409R00022